THE WELLNESS GUIDE

TIPS FOR CHOOSING THE BEST WELLNESS
PRODUCT FOR YOUR LIFESTYLE

KATE .P

Contents

CHAPTER ONE

INTRODUCTION

It's critical to select wellness goods that fit your lifestyle in order to preserve and improve your general well-being. The market is overflowing with a wide range of goods that make the claim to improve health and wellbeing, from beauty products and supplements to exercise gear and sleep aids. But without the right assistance, choosing the best items can be difficult. We'll go through important factors in this introduction to wellness product selection advice so you can make well-informed choices that suit your needs and interests.

Knowing Your Needs: Determining your individual health and wellbeing objectives is the first step towards selecting the appropriate wellness products. Whether your goals are to support general health, reduce stress, enhance skincare, or increase exercise, defining your goals can help you choose items that meet your needs.

Research and Education: Become knowledgeable about the components, advantages, and possible drawbacks of various wellness products by spending some time researching them. Seek reliable sources of data to learn about the safety and effectiveness of products, such as expert evaluations, scientific research, and consumer testimonials.

Safety and Quality: When choosing wellness goods, give priority to safety and quality. Select goods from respectable companies that use premium ingredients and strict quality control procedures. To guarantee the purity and efficacy of the product, look for third-party certifications such as Good Manufacturing Practices (GMP) or NSF International accreditation.

Ingredients and Formulation: Be sure wellness items satisfy your dietary and health needs by paying attention to their ingredients and formulation. Whenever feasible, choose products made with natural, organic, and non-toxic substances; stay away from goods with artificial additions, fillers, or allergens that could cause unfavorable reactions.

modification and Personalization: To meet your specific requirements and preferences, look for wellness goods that provide choices for modification and personalization. Customized vitamins, customized skincare routines, or customized exercise plans—all of these can be customized to meet your unique lifestyle and yield the best possible outcomes.

Consultation with Healthcare Professionals: For individualized advice, seek the advice of healthcare professionals including doctors, dietitians, or skincare specialists whenever in doubt. They may offer insightful advice based on your medical background, present state of health, and wellness objectives, assisting you in selecting the best items for your way of life.

Trial and Feedback: To determine whether a wellness product will fit into your lifestyle and preferences, try samples or smaller quantities before making a commitment. To get a variety of viewpoints, pay attention to how your body reacts to the product and ask reliable people for their opinions, such as friends, family, or online groups.

Utilizing these guidelines to select the ideal wellness goods for your way of life will enable you to confidently and wisely traverse the wide range of wellness offers. Whether you're starting a path toward improved fitness, beauty, or health, choosing the best goods suited to your needs will improve your quality of life and promote your general well-being.

The meaning of wellness products

A wide range of products intended to support mental, emotional, and physical well-being are referred to as wellness products. These products include a broad spectrum, such as healthy food and beverages, vitamins, beauty products, workout gear, tools for relaxation, and alternative therapies. Supporting and improving a person's overall health and wellness is the main goal of wellness products, which eventually helps people lead balanced and satisfying lives.

Important features of wellness products consist of:

Promotion of Health: By offering vital nutrients, antioxidants, vitamins, minerals, and other healthy substances that may be deficient in the diet or way of life, wellness products aim to enhance general health and wellbeing.

Health Issue Prevention and Management: A lot of wellness products are designed to help prevent or treat certain health issues, like vitamin deficiencies, inflammation, gastrointestinal issues, stress, anxiety, and sleep disturbances.

Natural and Holistic Approach: To promote wellness and vitality, wellness products frequently highlight a natural and holistic approach to health, including natural ingredients, botanical extracts, essential oils, and herbal medicines.

Personalization and customisation: To accommodate varying tastes, requirements, and health objectives, several wellness products provide personalization and customisation choices. This could involve nutritional advice, workout regimens, cosmetic products, and customized supplements.

Quality and safety are the most important factors to take into account while choosing wellness goods. Reputable companies use premium ingredients, strict quality control procedures, and extensive testing to guarantee the efficacy, potency, and purity of their products.

Accessibility and Convenience: Whether they are sold over-the-counter, online, or through medical professionals, wellness goods are usually made to be easy for customers to obtain and use. For the purpose of accommodating a range of tastes and lifestyles, they can be found in many formats, such as tablets, capsules, powders, lotions, oils, and gadgets.

Empowerment and Self-Care: By offering instruments, materials, and encouragement for self-care routines, wellness products enable people to actively participate in their own health and well-being. They promote self-awareness, self-compassion, and mindfulness as vital elements of a wholistic approach to wellbeing.

All things considered, wellness goods are crucial in assisting people in achieving and preserving their ideal levels of health, vitality, and quality of life. These items provide beneficial assistance for improving physical, mental, and emotional well-being, whether they are used as part of a regular wellness regimen or to address particular health issues.

Evaluating Individual Needs for Wellness

Examining your physical, mental, emotional, and social well-being as well as your social requirements will help you determine where you need to make improvements and create plans for improving your overall wellness. This process is known as "personal wellness needs assessment." You can evaluate your individual wellness needs by following these steps:

Self-Reflection: Give your present health and well-being some thought. Think about your emotional, mental, physical, and social well-being. Determine any areas that you could be struggling with, feeling uncomfortable, or not satisfied with.

Examine your medical history, taking into account any long-term illnesses, prior trauma, or inherited susceptibilities to particular diseases. Knowing your medical history can assist you in identifying possible risk factors and setting improvement priorities.

Physical Health Assessment: Examine your general level of fitness, food, exercise, and sleep quality when determining your physical health. Examine your sleep patterns, exercise routine, food choices, and any symptoms or medical concerns you may have.

Emotional and Mental Health Evaluation: Examine your emotional and mental health by considering your stress levels, resilience, mood, coping strategies, and general mental health. Think about any emotional imbalance, stress, worry, or depression that might be harming your health.

Assess your social networks, relationships, and support systems as part of your social health assessment. Think about how well you get along with your friends, family, coworkers, and neighbors. Determine whether your interactions with other people make you feel fulfilled, supported, and socially connected.

Establish Wellness Goals: Determine particular wellness objectives that are in line with your priorities, values, and aspirations based on your self-evaluation. Think about establishing objectives for stress management, relationship building, mental resilience, physical activity, nutrition, and personal development.

Seek Professional Guidance: To acquire more understanding of your wellbeing requirements and create individualized improvement plans, think about consulting with medical specialists, such as physicians, dietitians, psychologists, or wellness coaches. They can offer professional guidance, encouragement, and materials catered to your own wellness and health objectives.

Create a Wellness Plan: Create a thorough wellness plan that details the precise actions, behaviors, and strategies you will use to meet your wellness needs based on your assessment and goals. Make a schedule for when your goals will be implemented and break them down into doable phases. Think about combining a range of wellness techniques, such as self-care, social interaction, mindfulness, stress management, exercise, and healthy eating.

Track Your Progress and Make Adjustments: Keep a close eye on how well you're doing in terms of reaching your wellness objectives, and tweak your plan as necessary. Keep a record of your experiences, obstacles, and victories as you go. Remain adaptive and flexible, and be prepared to change your strategy in response to criticism and evolving conditions.

Exercise Self-Compassion: Keep in mind to treat your journey toward healing with kindness, tolerance, and self-compassion. Recognize that change may need time and work, and practice self-compassion while navigating the highs and lows of your own personal development.

You can develop a better, more contented, and well-balanced life by identifying your own wellness needs and acting to meet them. Make self-care a priority, pay attention to your body and mind, and make decisions that will benefit your general health.

Making a budget and defining priorities are the first steps in selecting the best wellness products for your needs. Here's how to budget and prioritize wellness product purchases:

Establish Your Wellness Goals: Establish your main aims for wellness and health. Are you concentrating on resolving certain health issues, stress management, skincare, or fitness enhancement? You can prioritize the wellness products that best suit your needs by making your goals clear.

Prioritize: After determining your wellness objectives, arrange them according to priority.

CHAPTER TWO

Think about the health and well-being issues that are most important or have the most effects on your overall quality of life. This will enable you to more wisely devote your funds to the things that are most important to you.

Allocate Funds Appropriately: Examine your spending plan and distribute funds in accordance with your priorities. Decide how much you can and will spend each month or year on wellness items. Think about designating a certain amount of your spending plan for costs related to your health and well-being.

Put Essentials First: Give top priority to wellness essentials that will help you achieve your main aims and objectives. These could be vitamins, necessary skincare products, workout gear, and tools for relaxation that help with particular health issues or promote your general wellbeing.

Investigate Product Options: Look into wellness items that satisfy your requirements regarding cost, effectiveness, and quality. Seek out trustworthy firms with merchandise that fits your spending limit and priorities. To make well-informed judgments, research possibilities, compare costs, and read reviews.

Think About Long-Term Value: Assess the wellness items' relative long-term value to their purchase price. Certain products might cost more up front, but they might end up saving more in the long run. When making purchases, think about choosing goods that will help your health in the long run and are within your means.

Investigate Cost-Saving Techniques: Seek out methods to cut costs on wellness supplies without compromising on quality. Take advantage of deals and promotions, buy in bulk, use coupons or discount codes, look into generic or less expensive brands, and use coupons or discount codes.

Set Boundaries and Limits: To avoid overspending on wellness goods, set boundaries and limits. Stick to your budget by deciding how much you're willing to spend on different products or categories. To keep within your limits, resist the need to make impulsive purchases and, if required, reevaluate your priorities.

Track Expenses and Make Adjustments: Maintain a record of all the money you spend on wellness and make sure you keep an eye on your spending. Periodically review your budget to see if your spending is in line with your priorities and make any necessary adjustments. Remain adaptable and prepared to reallocate money in response to evolving requirements and situations.

Practice Mindful Consumption: Make deliberate decisions about the wellness goods you buy and use to cultivate mindful consumption. Rather than giving in to marketing hype or trends, concentrate on things that truly help you and are consistent with your principles. Within your financial limits, you may maximize your investment in wellness and improve your general well-being by making thoughtful decisions.

You can choose wellness goods that promote your health and well-being while remaining within your financial means by prioritizing your needs and creating an effective budget. To establish a lasting and well-rounded approach to wellness, make sure your purchases are in line with your objectives, values, and financial constraints.

Aspects of Safety and Quality to Consider

Prioritizing quality and safety when selecting health products for your lifestyle is essential to ensuring that the items you choose are safe, dependable, and effective. The following are important quality and safety factors to remember:

Reputation and Brand Reliability: Select wellness products from brands that have a solid track record of manufacturing high-quality, safe, and efficient products. These brands are reliable and reputable. To determine a brand's legitimacy and dependability, look into its reputation, credentials, and client testimonials.

Third-Party Testing and Certification: To ensure the quality, safety, and purity of wellness products, look for those that have passed third-party testing and certification. Verification of product quality and adherence to industry standards can be obtained through certifications from respectable organizations like ConsumerLab.com, NSF International, and USP (United States Pharmacopeia).

Transparency and Disclosure of Ingredients: Give preference to wellness products that offer thorough and transparent ingredient lists that detail the source, potency, and purity of each ingredient. Steer clear of items with proprietary or unknown blends that are opaque about their dosage and composition.

Natural and Organic Ingredients: Whenever feasible, use wellness items made with non-toxic, natural, and organic ingredients. Seek certifications such as EcoCert, Non-GMO Project Verified, or USDA Organic to make sure the products fulfill strict requirements for sustainability and purity.

Avoiding Hazardous additions and Fillers: Examine the ingredient list for any artificial colors, flavors, preservatives, allergies, fillers, or additions that could be damaging to your health. Make sure to select items with little or no additives and give preference to clean, simple ingredient combinations.

Allergen Considerations: Carefully read product labels to identify any possible allergens if you have known allergies or sensitivities to specific substances. To prevent negative reactions, select wellness items devoid of common allergies including gluten, dairy, soy, nuts, and shellfish.

Compliance with Good Manufacturing Practices (GMP): To guarantee quality, consistency, and safety standards throughout the production process, be sure wellness products are made in facilities that follow GMP guidelines. Seek for goods with quality seals or GMP certifications visible on the packaging.

Dosage and Usage instructions: To prevent overusing or misusing wellness products, adhere to the manufacturer's recommended dosage and usage instructions. Be mindful of any cautions, restrictions, and possible drug interactions with pre-existing medical problems or prescriptions.

Consultation with Healthcare Professionals: For individualized guidance and recommendations, seek the assistance of healthcare professionals, such as physicians, pharmacists, dietitians, or herbalists, whenever in doubt. They can assist in determining the specific health needs you have, offer advice on appropriate products, and resolve any safety or efficacy issues.

Keep an eye out for any negative responses or side effects that you may have from health goods, such as gastrointestinal problems, allergic reactions, or symptom changes. If you encounter any negative side effects or have questions about the safety of the product, stop using it and get medical help.

When selecting wellness items for your lifestyle, you may make well-informed choices that promote your health and well-being without sacrificing efficacy or safety by giving quality and safety factors first priority. Make sure the goods you choose fit your needs and are consistent with your values by doing your homework, reading labels, and speaking with medical specialists.

Harmony with values and way of life

It's crucial to take your values, interests, and daily routines into account when choosing the best health items for your lifestyle. When determining whether a lifestyle and set of values are compatible, keep the following points in mind:

Personal Values and Beliefs: When selecting wellness goods, consider your own values, priorities, and beliefs. Think about how the items fit in with your beliefs about social responsibility, ethical sourcing, sustainability, cruelty-free procedures, and the environment.

Dietary Preferences and constraints: When choosing wellness goods, particularly food, drink, and supplements, keep your dietary preferences, constraints, and lifestyle decisions in mind. To be sure that the items fit your eating habits, choose those that cater to dietary choices like paleo, ketogenic, vegan, or vegetarian diets.

Fitness and Activity Level: When selecting wellness goods linked to physical activity and fitness, take into account your workout preferences, activity level, and fitness goals. To properly support your fitness journey, choose things that go well with your favorite exercise modalities, whether they be group fitness classes, weight training, yoga, running, or cycling.

Convenience and Accessibility: Consider how well-suited wellness items are to your daily schedule and way of life. Whether it's quick and easy to prepare meals, portable snacks, or space-saving home exercise equipment, pick things that are simple to include into your everyday routine.

Time Commitment and Sustainability: Determine whether using wellness products will fit into your schedule and lifestyle, as well as how much time it will take. Select items that are easy to use and long-lasting; stay away from excessively complicated or time-consuming choices that could not be viable in the long run.

Budget and Financial Considerations: When selecting wellness goods, keep your financial priorities and budget in mind. Choose items that fit within your budget and are reasonably priced; stay away from luxuries or needless expenditures that might not be necessary for your overall health.

Cultural and Ethnic Considerations: Take into account any cultural or ethnic influences on your product preferences and selections related to wellbeing. Whether it's herbal cures, conventional healing approaches, or culturally unique dietary preferences, choose products that speak to your cultural background, traditions, and practices.

Sustainability and Environmental Impact: Evaluate how wellness items will affect the environment and make eco-friendly, eco-conscious decisions. To lessen your environmental impact and encourage environmental sustainability, look for products with little packaging, recyclable materials, and sustainable sourcing methods.

Prioritize wellness goods that promote mental and emotional health, such as those that help with stress reduction, mindfulness, relaxation, and emotional resilience. To improve your overall quality of life, use goods that address the mind-body link and encourage holistic wellness.

Social Impact and Ethical Implications: Take into account the social impact and ethical implications of the companies and goods you decide to support. Choose goods from companies that uphold moral principles in business, exhibit social responsibility, and are dedicated to changing the world for the better.

You can choose wellness goods that promote your overall well-being and fit with your priorities and preferences by taking compatibility with your lifestyle and values into consideration. Select goods that improve your lifestyle, align with your ideals, and advance your general well-being.

Comprehending Marketing Claims and Products

It's important to comprehend marketing and product claims when choosing the best health items for your needs. It's critical to cut through marketing hype and find solutions that actually fit your demands because there are a lot of products on the market that make extravagant claims about how effective they are. The following are important things to keep in mind when interpreting product claims and marketing:

Be Wary of Overhyped promises: Wary of wellness items that make inflated or outlandish promises regarding their advantages. Look out for phrases like "quick fix," "miracle cure," or "guaranteed results," as they could be signs of deceptive marketing strategies.

Seek for Claims Supported by Research and Scientific proof: Look for wellness items that have research and scientific proof to back up their claims. On product packaging or marketing materials, look for references to clinical studies, peer-reviewed research, or scientific evidence. Products without reliable proof to support their claims should be avoided.

Distinguish Between Fact and Opinion: When assessing product claims, make a distinction between objective facts and subjective opinions. Anecdotal evidence and personal testimonials can offer valuable insights into product experiences, but they shouldn't be the only sources of information used to determine a product's efficacy.

Recognize Regulatory Oversight: Become acquainted with the rules and regulations pertaining to the claims made for wellness products in your area. For instance, the Food and Drug Administration (FDA) in the US controls dietary supplements and outlaws making deceptive or false claims. Seek for goods that abide by legal requirements and regulations.

Read Product Labels and Ingredients Lists Carefully: Learn what's in the product and how it might effect your health by carefully reading product labels and ingredient lists. Seek for transparent labeling procedures that make contents, dosage instructions, and any allergens readily apparent. Steer clear of items with opaque, proprietary blends that aren't revealed.

Be Wary of Marketing Gimmicks: Be wary of marketing gimmicks that could sway your opinion of a product, such as star endorsements, eye-catching packaging, or compelling advertising strategies. Pay more attention to the product's content than to its marketing gimmick.

Examine the Information Source: Take into account the reliability and objectivity of the sources that are offering advice on wellness items. To make well-informed selections, look for information from reliable sources, such as impartial review websites, scientific associations, and medical practitioners.

Consider Customer Reviews and Ratings: When evaluating the effectiveness and caliber of wellness goods, consider customer reviews and ratings. To obtain a fair picture, look for reviews from verified customers and take into account both good and bad comments.

Seek Accountability and openness: Select wellness brands that place a high value on accountability, openness, and moral business conduct. Seek out companies who are transparent about their sourcing, manufacturing procedures, quality control measures, and customer support guidelines.

Trust Your Instincts: When assessing wellness goods, rely on your gut feelings and intuition.

CHAPTER THREE

When buying a product, it's acceptable to move cautiously or look for further information if it seems too good to be true or raises red flags.

You can choose wellness items that support your values, lifestyle, and health objectives by being aware of product claims and marketing strategies. Remain watchful, conduct thorough study, and give preference to goods that provide openness, benefits supported by data, and veracity in their advertising.

Procedure for Trial and Evaluation

Finding the best health items for your lifestyle requires trial and error in order to assess their efficacy, compatibility, and fit for your specific requirements. To assist you in navigating the trial and evaluation process, below is a step-by-step guide:

Research and Selection: Begin by looking at several wellness items that fit your interests, lifestyle, and health objectives. Take into account elements including the components, claims made about the product, reviews, and advice from reliable sources. Reduce the number of items in your search to a select few that fit your requirements and look good.

Get Samples or Small amounts: If at all feasible, get samples or small amounts of the health items you're thinking about testing. This enables you to try the products before making a sizable initial investment.

Read the directions and guidelines carefully before using the products. The manufacturer has supplied usage guidelines, dosage recommendations, and instructions. To guarantee safe and appropriate use, heed any cautions, warnings, or contraindications.

Begin by Adding One Wellness Product at a Time: As you include each product into your routine, assess its impact and keep an eye out for any changes in your overall health and wellbeing. By beginning with a single product, you may more precisely evaluate its influence and steer clear of any possible interactions with other products.

Monitor Your Experience: Maintain a notebook or log to record your observations regarding any changes in your symptoms, vitality, attitude, or general state of well-being after using each wellness product. Keep track of any adverse effects, reactions to the product, and effects—both good and bad.

Track Short- and Long-Term impacts: Track the wellness products' impacts over time, both short- and long-term. While some products may show results right away, others might not show results until after using them consistently for several weeks or months.

Be Patient and Consistent: When conducting trials and evaluations, use patience and consistency. Allow enough time for each wellness product to do its job and refrain from passing snap decisions based on interim outcomes. Maintaining consistency is essential for precisely determining the items' efficacy.

Listen to Your Body: Observe how your body communicates with you and how the wellness products you're experimenting with affect it. When it comes to determining whether a product feels good for you and whether it's improving or worsening your health and wellbeing, follow your gut.

Get Input from Reliable Sources: Consult reliable sources who have used the wellness goods you're assessing, such as friends, family, medical professionals, or online groups.

Incorporating their viewpoints and thoughts into your assessment procedure is important.

Analyze Cost-Effectiveness: Consider the advantages, potency, and financial value of each wellness product when determining how cost-effective it is. Think about whether the product is worth adding to your long-term wellness routine and whether it yields noticeable results in relation to its price.

Make Well-Informed Decisions: Determine which wellness items are most advantageous and appropriate for your lifestyle based on your trial and evaluation process. Select goods based on your tastes, financial constraints, and health objectives.

Modify as Necessary: Remain open to modifying your wellness regimen in light of the conclusions you draw from the trial and assessment procedure. If a product isn't meeting your needs or is having unfavorable consequences, think about stopping its use and looking into more suitable solutions.

You may evaluate the efficacy and suitability of wellness items for your lifestyle and make well-informed decisions to promote your health and well-being by following these trial and assessment process steps.

Seeking Expert Advice

Getting professional help is a crucial step in selecting the best wellness items for your lifestyle, particularly if you require customized suggestions or in-depth knowledge. Here's how to successfully get expert advice while choosing health products:

Find Relevant Healthcare specialists: Based on your unique wants and concerns, ascertain which healthcare specialists would be most qualified to offer advice on wellness goods. Think about speaking with medical professionals, dietitians, pharmacists, herbalists, nutritionists, and naturopathic physicians.

Make Appointments: Make appointments with medical experts to go over your wellness product choices, worries, and health objectives. Make meetings with experts in fields related to your needs, like skincare, herbal medicine, nutritional supplements, and nutrition.

Prepare Information and Questions: Prior to your appointment, make a list of inquiries and pertinent details you would like to go over with the medical specialist. Give specifics about your medical history, current medications, dietary preferences, lifestyle choices, and any wellness products you are thinking about or are interested in.

Be Open and Transparent: Discuss your goals, lifestyle choices, and health-related issues with the medical expert during the appointment. To help the expert make recommendations that are specifically customized to your needs, please share any pertinent information regarding your allergies, sensitivities, medical history, and preferences.

Talk About Product Options: Have a conversation with the medical expert regarding various wellness goods that could be appropriate for your requirements. Request recommendations that take into account your unique health profile, clinical experience, and available scientific data.

Analyze Risks and Benefits: Consider the advantages and disadvantages of every wellness product that was mentioned in the consultation. Talk about any side effects, drug interactions, and contraindications to make sure the items are suitable for your health and safe.

Provide clarity on Dosage and Usage rules: Ask the healthcare provider to provide details on recommended dosages, usage rules, and any particular instructions needed to use the wellness items in an efficient manner. For best results, make sure you know how to include the products into your regular regimen.

Examine Alternatives and Complementary Therapies: Consult a healthcare provider about alternative wellness items or complementary therapies that could enhance your main course of therapy. Talk about the possible benefits of mixing various products or approaches for all-encompassing wellness support.

Request Follow-Up and Monitoring: Inquire with the medical practitioner about scheduling follow-up visits or having your progress monitored so that your wellness routine can be modified as necessary. Arrange for routine check-ins to talk about any changes in your symptoms, state of health, or reaction to the goods.

Remain Informed and Involved: Remain informed and involved when looking for expert advice on which wellness items to buy. Make sure the decisions you're making are in line with your values and health goals by actively participating in discussions, asking clarifying questions, and making in-depth inquiries.

You can get individualized recommendations, professional assistance, and evidence-based information to assist you in selecting the best wellness items for your lifestyle by consulting with healthcare professionals. Work together with experts who can support you in making decisions that will maximize your well-being and who are aware of your particular health needs.

Accepting a Holistic Perspective on Health

When choosing the best wellness items for your lifestyle, adopting a holistic perspective on wellness is essential. A holistic approach takes into account how many facets of health and wellbeing such as the mental, emotional, social, and spiritual are interconnected. The following are some ways to use a holistic viewpoint while selecting wellness products:

Evaluate Your Total Well-Being: To begin, evaluate your total well-being in terms of several aspects, such as your physical and mental health, your emotional and mental stability, your social life, and your spiritual fulfillment. Determine your areas of strength and those that might need more help or development.

Establish Holistic Wellness Objectives: After completing your assessment, make goals for your physical, mental, emotional, social, and spiritual well-being. Think about objectives like bettering your diet, controlling your stress, getting better sleep, building meaningful connections, and promoting personal development.

Think About Whole-Person Wellness: Select wellness items that promote overall wellness and concurrently address several aspects of health. Seek for goods that address all aspects of wellbeing rather than just one, such as those that aid the mind, body, and spirit.

Prioritize Balance and Prevention: Give top priority to wellness items that support balance and prevention in your general health and wellbeing. Look for goods that enhance the body's natural healing abilities, guard against sickness, and encourage balance and harmony in all facets of life.

Include Mind-Body Practices: To encourage holistic well-being, include mind-body practices in your wellness regimen. Select products that promote activities that improve physical, mental, and emotional resilience, such as breathwork, yoga, tai chi, qigong, mindfulness, and meditation.

Nourish Your Body with Nutrient-Dense Foods: Put your attention toward providing your body with foods high in nutrients to promote optimum health and vigor. To nourish your body and advance general health, choose whole, unprocessed foods high in vitamins, minerals, antioxidants, and phytonutrients.

Support Mental and Emotional Health: Make your choice of wellness products that improve mood, emotional resilience, and mental and emotional health by lowering stress and encouraging relaxation. Think about items like stress-relieving pills, aromatherapy oils, herbal teas, and relaxation aids.

Build Meaningful Relationships: Build relationships and meaningful connections that support your social and emotional health. Select wellness goods that promote community involvement, healthy social connections, and communication and connection with loved ones.

Maintain an Active Lifestyle: As part of your overall wellness regimen, make regular physical activity a priority and stay active. Select wellness products whether they be fitness monitors, workout gear, or exercise equipment that help you reach your fitness objectives and inspire movement.

Listen to Your Intuition and Inner Wisdom: When choosing wellness goods that support your overall well-being, follow your gut and your inner guidance. Make decisions that promote your general health and vitality and are consistent with your values by paying attention to your body's signals, emotions, and instincts.

By adopting a holistic perspective on health and taking into account the interdependence of the mind, body, and spirit, you may choose wellness items wisely to enhance your overall well-being. Select items that support your values, objectives, and lifestyle choices, then incorporate them into a holistic wellness regimen that supports your general well-being and vigor.

Summary

To sum up, choosing the best wellness items for your lifestyle is a careful, customized process that takes into account a number of variables to support your general health and wellbeing. These pointers can help you make well-informed decisions and select goods that suit your needs, tastes, and values:

Assess Your Needs: To choose the wellness products that will best support your well-being, start by evaluating your lifestyle, preferences, and health goals.

Investigate Various Wellness Products in-depth: Read up on the components, effectiveness, safety, and reliable sources' reviews of each product.

Seek Professional Advice: For individualized advice and recommendations catered to your unique health profile, speak with medical professionals or wellness specialists.

Think About Holistic Well-Being: When selecting items, use a holistic mindset and take into account how physical, mental, emotional, social, and spiritual components of health are interconnected.

Assessing Safety and Quality: Give top priority to goods that adhere to strict guidelines for safety, transparency in sourcing, manufacturing, and labeling processes.

Trust Your Instincts and Pay Attention to Your Body's Signals: When experimenting with new wellness items, pay attention to how they make you feel overall.

Remain Adaptive and Flexible: As your needs and tastes change over time, don't be afraid to try new items and modify your wellness regimen.

Spend Smartly: Set aside money for wellness products that best suit your health objectives and provide the greatest value.

Engage in Holistic Self-Care: Include wellness products in a self-care regimen that feeds your body, mind, and soul to support general health and energy.

Keep Yourself Educated and Empowered: Remain up to date on the most recent advancements in wellness goods, and give yourself the ability to make decisions that will benefit your long-term health.

You can improve your general health, vitality, and quality of life by adhering to these recommendations and making proactive decisions when selecting wellness items. Keep in mind that every person's path to optimum wellness is different, so follow your gut and give priority to goods that enhance your overall well-being and align with your values.

THE END